D0839813

EASY HEALTHCARE:

CHOOSING AN ASSISTED LIVING FACILITY

By

Lori-Ann Rickard

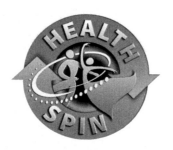

Presented by
Expert Health Press

To Dad who taught me everything I know.
You continue to inspire and support me.

TABLE OF CONTENTS

INTRODUCTION

As our loved ones age, we hope their lives will be comfortable and change will be minimal. There are very few of us who would choose to leave our home, where we have so many memories, and move to a place where we will live with and be taken care of by strangers. However, for many people, aging makes that choice necessary, when the need for care makes independence no longer possible.

If you or your loved one is considering moving to an assisted living facility, this guide is for you. Although I have spent over thirty years working in the healthcare industry, I knew next to nothing about assisted living facilities. Much of the recommendations in this guide are borne from "trial and error" for my own beloved father.

My dad was strong, smart and independent his whole life. He was a United Methodist minister who spent his entire life caring for others. He graduated from Albion College in Michigan and got his Doctorate of Divinity from Northwestern University. In addition to his church duties, he and my mother, a registered nurse, raised six children and watched more than seventeen grandchildren grow into adults. He preached about health and practiced what he preached every day by riding his bike, working out with weights, eating right, and almost always having a positive attitude about everything. As you can imagine, he NEVER saw his life including a move to an assisted living facility.

At eighty-eight years old, after living independently his whole life, my father underwent emergency back surgery, which caused him to lose his independence in one day. His procedure took place on April Fool's Day, and, due to his odd sense of humor, he thought that was a "perfect" day to change his life forever. As we maneuvered our way through the world of assisted living, he constantly asked what God was trying to teach him as he said growing old was the hardest thing he ever had to do.

Having been a healthcare lawyer for over twenty-seven years, I know a thing or two about healthcare. I also loved my dad as much as any daughter could. As the youngest of his six children, this was my chance to be his "rock," just as he had been mine all my life. What we both learned at every turn is that choosing an assisted living facility takes a lot of work, communication, and coordination. Most importantly, we found out that there is no perfect answer. This guide is for anyone who needs a "roadmap" like we did; a tool to consider much more than the obvious questions of location and cost.

So what are the 10 things you need to know when choosing an assisted living facility?

1.

PREPARATION: WHAT IS ASSISTED LIVING?

This may seem like a basic point, but when you begin to investigate senior living options, the list can quickly become confusing. However, it's important to know how each is different and what the best option is for your loved one. So, let's first establish just what "assisted living" is.

ASSISTED LIVING BRIDGES THE GAP

Assisted living facilities are the option that bridges the gap between **independent living** and **skilled nursing facilities** or **nursing homes**. You should consider an assisted living situation if your loved one can no longer live on their own, but does not require constant care or full-time medical care.

Assisted living facilities generally offer private living quarters where the resident can bring their own furnishings and decorations. Also, the staff will generally respect the resident's privacy and encourage independence and autonomy. Most residents live in the facility full time and their stay is unlikely to be temporary.

Seniors who do well in assisted living facilities often enter the facility at a younger age when they are still able to live somewhat independently. As a senior ages, the facility can add services to assist him or her. This is often referred to as "**aging in place.**" The senior may start by getting meals brought in to their apartment and possibly a cleaning service. As the senior's needs grow, services can be added. The senior might begin to need help with their medications or dressing and bathing themselves. There is no "one size fits all" but a menu of services that can be selected as the senior's needs increase. If the senior moves to the assisted living facility when they are very capable, the transition to increasing care is much easier. This is why it's helpful to start talking to your loved one as early as possible about assisted living options.

4

ACTIVITIES OF DAILY LIVING

An assisted living facility generally assists their residents with "**activities of daily living**," also known as ADLs. ADLs can include dressing, bathing, going to the bathroom, grooming, medications, and meal preparation. Your loved one may not always need this kind of assistance, but it is there when they need it. Most assisted living facilities offer communal living with housekeeping and laundry, planned activities, transportation, and exercise and wellness programs. There will likely be opportunities to gather with the other residents in the facility. Cable television and phone service is also available.

MEDICAL CARE WITHIN LIMITS

While most assisted living facilities will have a nurse who is in charge of medications, the nurse will not be in the facility 24/7. An aid will likely give the resident his or her medication if necessary. If the patient has a life-threatening problem, the facility will likely call 911. The facility may also have a therapy service that will come on site to provide physical or occupational therapy services to the residents who have a doctor's order for the therapy. **Medicare** and most insurance policies have a limitation on how much therapy a resident can get in a certain time period. Without a doctor's order, the facility may offer exercise classes but not with a licensed therapist.

Many facilities also offer special units for Alzheimer and dementia patients. The residents in the Alzheimer/Dementia units usually are located together, eat together, and have activities together for security and safety reasons. Because these special units often have a higher staff-to-resident ratio, a room in the Alzheimer unit will likely cost more than a regular room.

FOCUS ON INDEPENDENCE

Most good assisted living facilities focus on as much independence as possible for their residents. Your loved one is generally free to pursue his or her own interests and keep his or her own schedule. If the facility has a lot of rules and regulations about when your loved one can have visitors and when they can leave the facility, you should make sure this is a good "fit" for your loved one. It is often easier for the facility to have all the residents in the facility, for example, when the nurse or physical therapist finds it convenient to see the residents. If your loved one wants to continue their outside scheduled activities, make sure the facility will not limit them. The facility should be willing to accommodate what is best for your loved one.

MOVING ON FROM ASSISTED LIVING

You should know that there might come a time when your loved one is no longer allowed to live in the assisted living facility because he or she requires more full-time medical care. Some facilities will allow your loved one to stay; however, other facilities will likely talk to you about moving to another facility. Some facilities, on the other hand, will simply send you an eviction notice, which can be quite disturbing. Generally, the facility contract will allow administrators to give your loved one thirty days notice if they want him or her to leave. Thirty days is often not enough time to arrange for a move to a different facility. So, you should meet with the facility staff to determine a time frame that will meet everyone's needs.

PAYING FOR ASSISTED LIVING

Another major difference between different types of facilities is which insurance they will accept. Normally, only skilled nursing facilities and nursing homes accept Medicare, **Medicaid**, or private insurance. Most assisted living facilities only accept private pay. If your loved one has **long term care insurance**, you should check with the assisted living facility and the long term care insurance company to determine how such insurance is handled. It is likely that your loved one will have to make the monthly payment and get reimbursed by the long term care insurance company.

THE BOTTOM LINE...

- Before choosing this option for your loved one, know what "assisted living" means.

- Assisted living facilities are the option that bridges the gap between independent living and skilled nursing facilities or nursing homes.

- Assess your loved one's capabilities and future needs to decide if assisted living is the right fit for him or her.

- Assisted living facilities provide a variety of services for residents who need occasional assistance with "activities of daily living" (ADLs), which could include bathing, going to the bathroom, and taking medication.

- Assisted living facilities should focus on providing as much independence to your loved one as possible.

- If your loved one requires constant medical care, he or she will likely have to leave the assisted living facility for another facility, such as a nursing home.

2.

Preparation: What Assisted Living is NOT

Beyond assisted living, a range of senior care options exist that vary widely in their levels of care and cost. Depending on what your loved one needs, one of these options may be a better fit.

REHABILITATION FACILITIES

When a senior is temporarily unable to return to his or her current living situation after a hospital stay, a **rehabilitation facility** is often the next logical stop. A rehabilitation facility assists your loved one with regaining his or her strength and movement. A rehabilitation facility will have twenty-four-hour licensed or registered nursing staff and a physician who supervises each patient's care.

Care in a rehabilitation facility can include physical and speech therapy and occupational rehabilitation. The facility can also provide intravenous therapy, post-surgical stabilization, wound care, and pulmonary management. The rehabilitation facility will also provide the resident with bathing, grooming, dressing, and toileting. Since the living quarters are temporary, there is less ability for your loved one to have private living quarters that can be decorated with their possessions.

NURSING HOMES AND SKILLED NURSING FACILITIES

Next, compare an assisted living facility to a traditional nursing home or skilled nursing facility. A nursing home is generally certified by your state and provides 24/7 nursing care. Nursing homes provide round-the-clock medical care for all residents. Your loved one will likely need a nursing home if he or she is bed bound, on a respirator, has wounds that are not healing, or needs daily nursing care. Not surprisingly, nursing homes generally have residents with complex medical needs.

CONTINUING CARE RETIREMENT COMMUNITIES

At some facilities, called **continuing care retirement communities,** there will be independent living options, assisted living options and nursing home options. In rare cases, these facilities will also have an affiliation with a hospital. These facilities allow your loved one to start off in independent living and transfer to higher levels of care as it becomes necessary. If he or she is hospitalized for some reason, your senior will be discharged to the care level that best meets his or her needs at that time. These facilities offer the most flexibility for your loved one; however, they are often rare and difficult to find in every location.

SENIOR COMMUNITIES

Senior communities are essentially large facilities that house seniors in an independent living setting. These facilities may or may not offer some limited joint activities and services. For example, your loved one may be able to get some or all of their meals delivered to his or her apartment or eat in a common dining area. There may be activities offered for socializing with other residents. However, your loved one will basically be living independently. If there is a problem, the senior community will likely have you call 911. These facilities are recommended for seniors who are relatively healthy and enjoy engaging with others their age.

Some senior communities offer additional services through outside companies such as cleaning, visiting nurses, etc. These services will not be offered or supervised by the senior community staff so you should investigate these services separately from the facility.

RESIDENTIAL CARE HOMES

A residential care home is generally a private home where seniors live together and receive care by live-in caregivers. Residents are generally provided assistance with ADLs such as grooming, dressing, bathing, etc. All of their meals are prepared for them; however, they generally eat together with the other residents, not in their individual rooms. The home may provide other services such as a visiting nurse or physical therapy depending on what the resident's doctor orders. These types of homes vary widely so it is very important to do your "homework" on any residential care home you are considering.

THE BOTTOM LINE...

- Rehabilitation facilities allow for short-term stays generally after a hospitalization.

- Nursing homes house residents with complex medical needs who require constant medical care.

- Senior communities offer independent living options, but very few services to assist with activities of daily living.

- Continuing care retirement communities offer graduated levels of care from independent living to nursing home care; however, these facilities are rare.

- Residential care homes are private homes where seniors live together and have live-in care. The quality of residential care homes will vary greatly since each is run differently based on the skills and approach of the private owner.

3.

PREPARATION: ENGAGE YOUR LOVED ONE NOW

When selecting an assisted living facility, the most important thing you can do is involve your loved one in as many decisions as possible during the process. However, this is often easier said than done. Everyone wants to avoid difficult conversations, and many people as they age resist discussing something as life-changing as a move, especially when that move may represent "surrendering" to old age.

Additionally, your loved one may be unable to properly evaluate his or her needs. You may notice changes in health and well-being that he or she does not. They may be isolated and depressed. You may notice he or she is not regularly changing their clothes and can no longer keep up with household chores. You might notice that he or she is forgetting daily medications.

This is why the earlier you start to have this discussion, the better, ideally before he or she is no longer able to live independently. Talk with your loved one about where other people his or her age are living. When his or her friends move, take your loved one to visit so he or she can evaluate the positives and negatives of the facility. The more you approach this as a joint decision, the easier the decision will be. Have your loved one read this guide and other useful information so he or she can become informed.

CONSIDER WHERE YOUR LOVED ONE CURRENTLY LIVES

Is it a large, single family home? Is it a condominium? Is it a second-floor apartment with lots of stairs? When your loved one must start downsizing his or her life, it is important to be a partner in deciding what the next steps should be, both long term and short term. For example, if he or she is selling the family home as an "empty nester," a small, ground-floor apartment or a ranch-style condominium may be the logical next step for someone who is currently independent, but who may need to use a cane or a wheelchair in the future. Or they may want to live in the social setting of a senior community. However, depending on the situation, the level of care your loved one requires may make these more independent situations unrealistic.

MAKE A LIST OF WHAT IS MOST IMPORTANT

Key to selecting an assisted living facility is sitting down with your loved one and determining what is most important for his or her new living environment. Does your loved one have extensive healthcare needs? Is a private room important? What are your loved one's likes and dislikes? What is his or her social disposition? This list will evolve as you start to tour facilities and learn more about the options. Many assisted living facilities may have services that your loved one will never take advantage of. The staff at my dad's assisted living home took pride in having a wide variety of activities for the people who lived there. My dad, however, was a very private man, and at eighty eight, was not going to start attending social hour, flower arranging classes, or bingo. Other residents, however, looked forward to such events. So, knowing what your senior enjoys and what he or she will not care about helps in choosing an assisted living facility.

What locations are you going to consider? If you have family spread all over the country, where should you look? Some seniors would like to stay in the location where they have lived their whole life. Others would prefer to move to a warm climate. Is there a family member who has more time than others to devote to helping your loved one? All of these are important things to consider when making your list of priorities.

WHAT BELONGINGS WILL YOUR LOVED ONE TAKE TO THE ASSISTED LIVING FACILITY?

No matter how large the rooms or apartments are at potential assisted living facility, it is likely that your loved one will be unable to take everything he or she has acquired over their many years. In fact, if your loved one needs to save on costs by sharing a room, he or she will have even less room for things from home. Once you've started the conversation about assisted living, it's important for your loved one to think about what personal items are most important to keep with them.

Factors to consider include what will happen to his or her current home. Will it be sold? Will another family member live there? Will your loved one's current belongings be stored or sold? Will some be given away to other family members? All of these discussions are difficult, but important to know for the move. If possible, do not sell your loved one's home immediately upon his or her move to an assisted living facility (if he or she does not currently live in an apartment). It generally helps to allow for a period of adjustment when your loved one does not have to learn to live in a new environment while at the same time packing up or selling his or her belongings and knowing his or her home will be gone forever.

Many assisted living facilities offer to supply furniture for your loved one's room. Even if you use that furniture, it's often a good idea to take some furniture from your loved one's home. He or she is already going through a period of stressful change, and having a cherished piece of furniture will make the new room feel more like home. For my dad, it was his desk. Despite being far too big for his room, the desk would not accommodate his wheelchair and so it was nearly unusable. But it was the desk at which he had written many sermons and consoled many people as a beloved pastor. So we made this piece of home fit.

Another practical, but important, issue revolves around the assisted living facility's policy about putting things on the wall, painting the walls, etc. Pictures and mementos are important to making your loved one feel comfortable in his or her new room. Take those things that are most meaningful to your loved one. If they have a cherished item, bring it. Make the room look as close as possible to what they had at home. Take time to decorate the walls with things they love in the style they would want.

All of these discussions are important since downsizing is hard for anyone. It is especially hard when your loved one must also confront his or her loss of independence.

DOES YOUR LOVED ONE HAVE A WILL OR TRUST?

Another difficult, but necessary, conversation to have in advance with your loved one is to ensure that he or she has all of their affairs in order before entering an assisted living facility. If your loved one has not already executed a will or a trust, you should urge him or her to do so now. The documents should include a **durable power of attorney** and a **medical power of attorney**. Assuming your loved one is currently mentally competent, these documents need to be completed as early as possible so that if a medical emergency occurs and your loved one cannot communicate, his or her wishes will be followed.

These documents should identify who will have the ability to make decisions about your loved one's financial and medical issues. The documents should also designate whether your loved one wants everything done to prolong life in the case of an emergency or whether he or she wants to set limitations. For example, your loved one might want CPR if he or she stops breathing, but might not want to agree to extensive medical intervention such as being placed on life support.

YOUR LOVED ONE'S "BUY-IN" WILL MAKE THE ENTIRE PROCESS SMOOTHER

All of these recommendations regarding your loved one are meant to make the choice of an assisted living facility easier on everyone involved. It may be difficult to face talking to your loved one about this very stressful time in both your lives. However, the more you are open to a discussion and being a partner in the decision, the easier the choice will be.

Above all, remember that this move is not about "you." Avoid concentrating on how you feel about the move or the new facility and keep the focus on your loved one and what he or she is experiencing.

THE BOTTOM LINE...

- The more you engage your loved one and be his or her partner in the decision, the easier the choice will be.

- Evaluate where your loved one is currently living.

- Remember: There is "no place like home."

- Consider what belongings your loved one will take with them. Make the most important ones work in the new setting.

- Make sure your loved one has his or her legal affairs in order before moving to an assisted living facility.

- Remember: This move is not about you.

4.

Preparation: What Roles Will Family Members Have in Caring for Your Loved One?

Many families hope that the only challenge they will face will be to pick the right facility and then the ongoing care of their loved one will shift to the facility. Their only job will be to visit when convenient. However, this is rarely the case. And if that is how your family approaches your loved one's care, he or she will rarely be happy under those circumstances.

FAMILY COMMUNICATION IS KEY

An assisted living facility can certainly be of great help in caring for your loved one, but there is still much to do once he or she is a resident. It is extremely important that you discuss this openly with the other members of your family. This is, of course, another very difficult topic, but one that is essential to your loved one's well-being and your family's harmony. Often families avoid this topic, which leads to bad feelings and resentment as circumstances play out. Direct and open communication always works best, if possible. Also, recognize that issues will grow and change over time so a decision that is made today may need to be revisited in the future. Your loved one is aging and that brings new and different challenges over time.

WHO WILL BE THE "STUCKEE?"

While everyone says they want to "be there" for their loved one as they age, the task of being "on call" for whatever issues arise often falls to one person, the one "stuck" with all the problems. And no matter how much that family member wants to help his or her loved one, the many responsibilities can feel overwhelming.

So, from the outset, you should be asking: which family members will have what jobs? Will someone be the main contact for all issues? Or will you split responsibilities and have one person in charge of healthcare issues and another in charge of finances? Who will communicate with the facility when there are problems? How will your loved one get to doctor's appointments, church, and social engagements? Remember you are choosing an assisted living facility because your loved one wants to maintain some independence. How will your family or circle of friends assist your loved one with those things that he or she is unlikely capable of handling by themselves?

If one family member lives close to your loved one, is he or she the logical choice for being the primary caregiver? Or should you pick someone who might be unemployed or not currently working, as he or she would have more time to help? These are all decisions that vary from family to family and should be carefully considered. If you are going to divide up tasks, be certain that everyone involved communicates openly and regularly. If necessary, write down the division of responsibilities to make sure everyone clearly understands their role and how they will interact.

For instance, one family member might be local and in charge of issues that arise at the facility. Another family member who lives far away might be in charge of the finances. When the local family member determines that the level of care must be raised at the facility because their loved one has had a health setback, he or she must know what the financial status is in order to determine if paying for the higher level of care is possible. Both people must communicate to determine what is best. Often, these roles are blended, but the better the communication, the better care your loved one will receive.

Consider Compensating the Family Member Doing the Work

If one person will have the main responsibility of caring for your loved one, will he or she be paid? This is often a tough conversation to have as facility charges and medical bills put increasing pressure on the family's financial resources. To be sure, everything is more expensive than planned and resources are finite. But, assuming your family does have the resources, it might make sense to compensate the family member doing most of the work.

If your loved one is often in need of extra care or companionship beyond what the facility provides, it will likely be less expensive to pay a family member than to hire an outside agency to provide the extra care. Additionally, if you have a family member who is making a huge commitment of time and energy, your loved one may feel that compensating him or her from their own funds can be a way of expressing gratitude. Also, compensation may help the primary caregiver feel less resentful of the other family members who do not provide as much help.

If your loved one or your family does not have the resources to pay your loved one's primary caregiver, consider giving him or her something that might have value other than an hourly wage. For example, does your loved one own a home that might provide a place to live for the family member? Consider other items that your loved one might put in their will or trust that would compensate the family member after death. Was your loved one planning on contributing to one of the grandchildren's college fund? If so, maybe this contribution can be made as payment for the assistance your loved one needs. As is so often true in moving someone from independent living to assisted living, you must think "out of the box" to find solutions that aren't always obvious.

THE FACILITY WILL REQUIRE ONE FAMILY MEMBER TO BE THE CONTACT

If you have a large family, the facility will commonly ask that you select one person to be the primary person they will communicate with about your loved one. If that person is not the family member responsible for healthcare issues, communication is again key. It is understandable that the facility cannot be responsible for speaking to every family member about all aspects of care. The facility needs to know who to call when a problem arises.

Selecting one person in the family as the main point of contact does not mean that other family members are necessarily restricted from getting information about your loved one. If the issues are medical, the facility will likely require your loved one to designate who in the family can get medical information. Federal law requires that authorization be given to disclose medical information. The loved one can designate whomever he or she chooses. Unless the resident is mentally incompetent and has a guardian, the resident can choose everyone in the family, one person, or none.

It may be that one or many members of the family are paying for their senior's monthly assisted living facility charge. Because they are paying the bill, these family members may think they are automatically entitled to the senior's medical information. This is not true. No matter who is paying for the assisted living facility charges, the senior always maintains the right to have his or her healthcare information disclosed only to those people he or she chooses unless the senior is incompetent. If the senior is deemed by law to be incompetent, the guardian or trustee will have the right to authorize any and all disclosures.

HAVE A BACKUP

If you are selecting one family member to be in charge of most issues, your family should have a backup list of who can help if this person is out of reach, has his or her own emergency, or needs to take a deserved break from his or her caregiving responsibilities. Also, when your loved one has a health crisis, more care may be necessary for a temporary period. Consider having an agreement that the family members who live out of town will take rotations if your loved one has surgery or is hospitalized.

Because some family members may be unable to help due to other family commitments or work, it is also helpful to consider having a **nursing service** or **in-home care** service available for emergencies. When your loved one is ill, it can be a relief to know you have a trusted service available that can fill in the gaps when needed. If possible, research these services before you need them, and make sure you know what kind of nursing care is covered by Medicare and any gap insurance your loved one may have. Only consider nursing services that are licensed and bonded, get recommendations, and always check references. Good sources for recommendations include other families with seniors as well as your local hospital's discharge planners or social workers.

These services generally require some notice and have a minimum hourly requirement. Also, you should ask whether you can secure the same individual as often as possible. When your loved one is ill, having a friendly, known person is often very comforting.

THE BOTTOM LINE...

- Family communication is key! Set up conference calls or have face-to-face meetings with everyone involved.

- Decide whether one person will be in charge of all issues or whether the family will divide up tasks.

- Consider compensating the person who will handle most duties.

- The facility will require that the family select one person to communicate with.

- Have a backup for emergencies and life events so the family knows who to call when your senior needs extra help.

- Consider hiring a nursing service to cover the gaps when family members can't care for your loved one.

5.

PREPARATION: TAKE YOUR LOVED ONE TO TOUR VARIOUS ASSISTED LIVING FACILITIES

Touring prospective assisted living facilities with your loved one is a key step in making your decision. The best approach is to gather a list of local facilities or those in your loved one's target community, then gather basic information about each one to narrow down that list for actual visits. If, for example, a location is out of range financially, it's better to find that out before you take a tour and fall in love with the facility.

Remember that assisted living facilities are big businesses. Speaking to a representative of an assisted living facility is no different than talking to a real estate agent about buying a house. The sales people are likely being paid on commission and are incentivized to fill their facility with residents. When you contact an assisted living facility, they will want you to come in right away. Many facilities will tell you they "only have one room left." Remember the rule of "buyer beware." No one should make such a big decision feeling pressured. As much as possible, get any initial information in writing. Relying on verbal promises about costs and conditions is never a good approach.

Once you have done your homework, select two to three locations to tour with your loved one. The sooner you start this process the better. If your loved one has time to reflect on choices, the better the selection process will be for both of you. Obviously, emergencies can sometimes result in a sudden move. However, even a sudden hospitalization shouldn't automatically cause an immediate move to an assisted living facility. Medicare and most insurance plans will cover a thirty-day stay in a rehabilitation facility after a hospitalization, which will give you a longer period for you and your loved one to consider your choices.

As you tour the various facilities, make sure your loved one is engaged and involved in asking questions. After all, it is going to be their home so he or she should be as involved as possible. Spend time meeting other residents and their families, if possible. Have several meals at the facility so your loved one can sample what he or she would eat if they lived there. If the facility is owned by a parent company with a number of locations, make sure you investigate those other locations. Do not assume that each of their locations have the same set up, pricing, etc. Some locations have higher prices than others.

KEEP IN MIND: THERE'S NO PLACE LIKE HOME

As you are touring various facilities, keep your priority list handy, and remember that there are pros and cons to every living arrangement. However, one thing is for certain: you will simply not be able to replace your loved one's home. Nor will living at the facility be the same as living with family. This is a hard concept to grasp, as the facilities will never be what we want. Considering how much you must pay for an assisted living facility you would think that you could find one that is better than home. After all, most facilities provide meals, activities, and assistance with dressing, showering, if necessary. But most people find that no matter how lovely the place is – it is just not home.

What underlies this dissatisfaction is the reality that the time when your senior could take independence for granted is truly over. Every senior must try to make his or her own version of peace with the aging process. Not surprisingly, this takes time and much adjustment. It is better to recognize and come to terms with every new reality than to keep looking for something that does not exist. Nothing is perfect. If your loved one is really struggling with the changes in his or her health and living situation, always consider talking to his or her doctor, or bringing in a geriatric therapist.

When a senior is in the midst of moving to an assisted living facility, it's normal for him or her to become anxious or depressed. Symptoms may include becoming suddenly withdrawn, having a lack of interest in eating, or problems with sleeping. These symptoms should be monitored and may be best discussed openly with your loved one's doctor. It's also helpful to discuss these symptoms with your loved one rather than to ask if they are "depressed." Many seniors, like my dad, will not accept that they might be depressed, so it is much easier to talk about more objective issues such as appetite and sleep. A good primary care doctor who regularly works with seniors can be essential to helping your loved one through this process.

THE BOTTOM LINE...

- Gather a list of facilities in your loved one's target community. Then gather basic information (price, accommodations, etc.) on each one to narrow down that list for actual visits.

- Sales representatives at assisted living facilities are likely paid on commission and are incentivized to fill their facility with residents.

- Do not make a decision when feeling pressured.

- Get any initial information about the facility in writing.

- Meet current residents and their families.

- Eat several meals at the facility.

- Remember that no facility will be like home or living with family.

- During the selection process and after the move, monitor your loved one for signs of depression. Seek professional help if needed.

6.

MAKING THE DECISION:
START WITH THE BIG STUFF

So now that you and loved one have decided that an assisted living facility is right choice and you've done the work to prepare your family and loved one for the decision, what factors should you consider in selecting an actual facility? Let's start with the big stuff.

LOCATION, LOCATION, LOCATION

First, consider location. Is it nearby the family member who will be responsible for most of the care? Is it near the location where your loved one previously lived? Is it near places your loved one will want to go to regularly, such as their church, a beloved park, or the local coffee shop where their friends gather? Is the location easy for friends and family to get to? All of these factors should be prioritized and evaluated by you and your loved one when choosing from available assisted living facilities.

My dad grew up in a small town in Michigan. When he retired, he and my mom returned to that town to live. They reconnected with friends, family, and his childhood church, where he would serve as pastor emeritus. They lived close to the bike path they loved and the park they went to almost every day. And it was near my home and office. After my mother passed away and my father suddenly lost his independence, I became the one in the family primarily responsible for his care, so it made sense to move him into a facility near to me. I do have three brothers who could have cared for my father: one who lived an hour away and two others who lived on opposite coasts in California and Washington, D.C. However, it soon became clear that my dad did not want to move away from his friends, his church, and my family. So staying in Michigan near me became the only option.

We began our search for an assisted living facility near to my home; however, we ultimately chose a facility closer to my office than my home, a decision that turned out to be a smart one in the end. Normally, I'm at my office more than home, so if my father or the facility needed me, I was that much closer. Also, my office staff became my circle of support since my daughters were away at college and could only help out occasionally. If my dad had an emergency and I was out of town or could not be reached, one of my staff could stop by for a quick visit to handle the issue temporarily. Obviously not everyone has that option, but how location impacts your loved one's support network and your own is an important factor to consider when selecting an assisted living facility. Your support network may be your own children, your friends, or even your parent's younger siblings. Is the facility convenient to that network, or at least to the core? Can they get there when you can't?

HOW BIG IS THE FACILITY?

Next, consider the size of the assisted living facility. How many residents live there? Must your loved one walk down lots of long hallways to get to activities and meals? When the facility is very large and hundreds of other residents live there, it's generally more difficult to navigate, and, if your loved one has mobility issues, may present a problem. Also, meals will likely be more institutional at a facility that must feed a large amount of people three times a day. On the other hand, a large facility may offer a wider variety of activities and services as well as a greater opportunity for your loved one to make friends. As we have discussed, no perfect place exists, so you and your loved one must look to your list of priorities and determine which size is the best fit.

HOW MUCH DOES IT COST?

Cost is the next big consideration when choosing a facility. Since you don't know how long your loved one will be there, it's difficult to know what the total cost will be. Also, it's very important to ask about all potential costs, not simply the initial monthly fee. Before your loved one moves in, many locations will initially quote a relatively low fee, but once he or she is a resident and his or her abilities change, you may find out that many necessary services require additional fees. For example, if your mother can manage taking her medications on her own, the facility will likely quote you a basic level fee. But if she needs medication assistance later on, you will likely have to pay an additional fee. Those additional fees are often very high, so knowing them up front to help you plan for later on is important.

Some facilities will initially come to your loved one's home or hospital room to evaluate his or her needs and abilities. They might also ask you to fill out a questionnaire to assess what level of care your loved one will require. Different levels of care have different costs, so be clear and honest about your loved one's abilities. You don't want the facility to charge more than is necessary, but neither do you want to be surprised when costs suddenly go up after he or she has moved in and staff better understand his or her capabilities.

You also need to know if you must make an initial one-time deposit. Some facilities require this deposit to "join the community." Often non-refundable, this fee can be upwards of $5,000 or more. If the deposit is refundable, you should also ask whether your loved one is required to live at the facility for a certain amount of time before that fee can be returned. Also you should know how much notice you must give if your loved one does leave.

REVIEW ANY CONTRACTS BEFORE SIGNING THEM

The facility should have a standard contract for you and your senior to sign. Before signing, however, ask for a blank copy of the contract so you can review all of the costs and details before you make your final decision. Often circumstances force individuals to find a safe living arrangement for their loved ones in a hurry, and the tasks to complete seem endless. However, take the time to read the contract. Ask if you can negotiate any changes to the contract or fees involved. Most families have the difficult task of balancing cost with the preferred care their loved one wants and deserves.

Be a smart consumer before you make any commitment. It is not uncommon for the facility staff to tell you that they only have one room left and your deposit is required immediately to secure the room. Be wary of any "hard sell" tactics. The facility sales staff is often paid on commission and all facilities make the most when all the rooms are full. Take your time and make a thoughtful decision. Don't be rushed by anyone.

THE BOTTOM LINE...

- Consider location first. If at all possible, make sure you honor your loved one's wishes regarding location.

- If you are the one most responsible for your loved one's care, consider locations that are convenient for you and your support system.

- Use your list of priorities to determine if a large or small facility is best for your loved one.

- Ask to review all the costs, not just the monthly rate. Beware of hidden fees after you move in.

- Be honest about your loved one's abilities when determining levels of care.

- Be aware that you may have to pay a deposit up front.

- Review all contracts before signing them. Do not be pressured to sign a contract on the spot.

7.

THE MOST IMPORTANT QUESTION: WHO ARE THE STAFF?

No question regarding an assisted living facility is as important as this. Staff members are the front line in caring for your loved one, and their skills, attitude, and abilities will have real impact on your loved one's health and quality of life.

STAFF-TO-RESIDENT RATIO AND RESPONSE TIMES

The first question to ask is: what is the ratio of staff to residents? The amount of staff per residents is important for many reasons. The more staff the facility has the more residents they are able to serve at a time. Most facilities have one staff member for every six to eight residents. The ratio will be higher during the nighttime hours, with often one staff member caring for fifteen residents.

It's important for you and your loved one to understand that no assisted living facility will offer one-to-one care. In practical terms, this means that your loved one will likely notify the staff that they need assistance by ringing a bell or pushing a button (in a very small facility, the patients might just call for the staff by name). Responsible assisted living facilities have clear requirements for staff to respond in a maximum pre-determined amount of time. A typical reasonable timeframe during the day is ten minutes, but that time will likely be longer at night.

Given that it will dictate how long your loved one will wait until, for example, they can be taken off the toilet, it is important to know what the system is for contacting the staff for assistance and how that system will be monitored. If the facility uses a computerized system, supervisors should be able to easily generate statistics regarding response times. Also, facilities are often chronically understaffed so ask what the actual ratio of staff-to-residents is at the facility where your loved one will live. And ask for actual response times. Do not accept "general" averages or averages across facilities if the residence is part of larger corporation.

Also ask questions about the age, reliability, and maintenance of the paging system used by patients to notify staff. It's common for the paging system to fail or be unreliable. This is an important question to ask when considering a facility; if the paging system fails, your loved one will have no way of contacting the staff in an emergency.

Make sure that staff and administrators will be open to negotiating response times for your loved one when it makes sense. You can imagine that waiting will be one of the greatest frustrations for him or her after moving into the facility. Previously independent, your loved one must now wait to get dressed, wait to get bathed, wait to eat, and more. Moreover, the bigger the facility, the greater the frustration will be. For example, if staff members have eight other residents to care for and your loved one needs assistance getting to the dining room, he or she will often have to wait until seven other people are seated.

While waiting is an unavoidable aspect of assisted living, competent staff will be responsive to working with you and your loved one to minimize wait times in some circumstances. My dad for example, was an early riser. He liked to get up, get dressed, and have breakfast. We had to meet several times with the facility to change the order of their duties to accommodate his needs. When you have a facility that is eager to make the resident comfortable, you can usually work through these issues.

STAFF TRAINING AND EXPERIENCE

You should also ask about staff training, education, and experience. Resident caregivers are often high school graduates. Some have a level of training or certification in a healthcare discipline, but not all. Ask what sort of ongoing training staff members receive at facility. Also ask what their education requirements are for hiring caregivers. Also, if caregivers speak English as a second language, can they be easily understood by the residents? This seems like a silly question; however, it can be very frustrating (and potentially harmful) for your loved one if he or she cannot communicate with a staff member who is otherwise completely capable of providing care.

It is also very important to ask how much turnover the facility has. It is not uncommon for staff members to come and go, as caregiving positions tend to be entry-level jobs. However, a high rate of turnover can be a red flag that the facility administrators do not create an atmosphere where competent employees want to stay. Additionally, find out if the facility makes an effort to have the same caregivers with the same residents as often as possible. If your loved one can establish a rapport with some of the caregivers, they will feel more comfortable than if there is always someone new.

STAFF ATTITUDE

Also, observe the staff when they are working with other residents. Are they taking the time to talk to the residents, or just rushing to get done with a task and leave? Do they seem genuinely interested in the residents? Do they speak warmly to the residents or are they gruff? Do they pay more attention to their phone than to residents? What is the relationship between staff and administrators? Are competent, high-performing staff rewarded?

Take the time to see staff in action before choosing a facility. These are the people who will care for your loved one every day and have the greatest impact on his or her well being. It is important that the facility stresses the importance of the caregivers' relationship with the residents, not just how efficient they are.

THE BOTTOM LINE...

- Find out what the staff-to-resident ratio is.

- Know that no assisted living facility will provide one-to-one care.

- Know the time it takes for staff to respond to residents when called. Make sure the facility is open to negotiating response times when appropriate.

- Understand the system for calling staff.

- Ask about staff training, education, and experience.

- Ask about staff turnover. Facilities with high turnover may not be able to retain quality caregivers.

- Observe the attitude of the staff. Make sure they are engaged and interested in caring for their residents.

8.

MEDICAL EMERGENCY POLICIES

Obviously, you and your loved one are considering a move to an assisted living facility because you believe he or she will be safe and well cared for there. However, when it comes to medical emergencies, it's not always clear what a facility's policies and procedures are.

WHO CALLS 911?

First, ask if the facility has a written policy for handling emergencies. If they have one, ask for a copy. Is the policy simply to call 911? Is your loved one responsible for calling 911? Or, does the facility have medical staff that performs CPR and other basic life-saving techniques?

If the facility merely asks your loved one to call 911, make sure he or she is comfortable with that scenario. If your loved one is not comfortable, but you want to keep the facility on your list for other reasons, you might also want to consider purchasing your loved one a **personal emergency alert device** to wear so he or she can easily call for help if they fall or have a medical emergency.

WHICH HOSPITAL?

In the event of a medical emergency, will your loved one be taken from that facility to the hospital best for him or her? An ambulance arrives at an assisted living facility one of two ways: the facility staff will either directly call the ambulance service they have a contract with or they will call 911 and a local ambulance will be dispatched. In most states, the ambulance by law must take your loved one to the nearest appropriate hospital, which may not be where his or her doctors practice. If it is not, your loved one will likely be assigned an "on call" doctor who is unfamiliar with your loved one's medical history and unlikely to have immediate access to their medical records.

If being at a particular hospital is important, you should consider this when selecting an assisted living facility. Transferring to another hospital after admission is often difficult depending on your loved one's condition. Alternatively, if you choose a specific assisted living facility near a specific hospital, you may want to choose physicians who are on staff at that hospital to take regular care of your loved one.

WHAT IF YOUR LOVED ONE NEEDS NON-EMERGENCY CARE?

When evaluating an assisted living facility, find out how they intend to work with you and your loved one in determining when your senior needs medical care. Whenever possible, you want to contact your loved one's doctor to determine if a trip to the emergency room is necessary, since that trip is often very expensive and time-consuming. Many times, a health issue can be resolved with a visit to the primary care doctor if identified early on.

Staff at a well run assisted living facility will know to communicate to residents' loved ones early in the day, preferably on a weekday, if they see signs that he or she might need medical attention. They know that waiting to alert you to symptoms until after hours or the weekend means that your loved one's likely only option for care is the emergency room. Also, make sure the facility will check with you as symptoms worsen. No one wants to get a call from the facility after the ambulance has already arrived.

THE BOTTOM LINE...

- Make sure you know whether the facility will contact 911 for an emergency or if your loved one must call instead.

- Consider purchasing your loved one a personal emergency alert device.

- Make sure you know which hospital your loved one will be transported to in case of an emergency.

- Consider switching doctors if they are not on staff at the hospital closest to the facility.

- Chose a facility that will work with family to identify early on when a senior needs nonemergency medical care.

9.

THE SMALL STUFF THAT'S NOT SO SMALL: WHAT'S A DAY LIKE?

Location, cost, staff, and medical policies are among the "big" deciding factors in choosing an assisted living facility. However, there are plenty of "small" things that in reality may be the most important to your loved one. Always remember that this is where your loved one is coming to live, and he or she may be there for a very long time. The assisted living facility will be so much more than an institution providing housing and medical care. It is the next phase of "home" for your loved one. So you should ask: What will my loved one's day be like? What is the quality of activities and meals? How much of your loved one's previous life can he or she live?

What Is the Schedule?

Your loved one's schedule provides great comfort. When do I get up? When do I bathe? How often is my laundry done? Who will help me get dressed? When is breakfast, lunch, and dinner? What activities are available in the morning and afternoon? Does the facility have transportation for getting to and from those activities? Who can visit and when? Every facility is different so understand the flow of the ones on your list.

Many facilities allow family and friends to come and go as they like and treat the resident's room as his or her own. Other facilities have strict visiting hours. If your loved one is sick or simply needs some company, can a family member stay in the room with them overnight? Again, if this is important to you, make sure you know the facility's policy up front. Additionally, you should also find out if your loved one can freely come and go from the facility, assuming he or she is capable of doing so safely.

Will the facility work with residents to go to or arrange activities they might suggest or be interested in? For example, my very independent father disliked planned activities and refused to participate unless coaxed. However, he loved sports, and he soon found out that the executive director of his facility played in a hockey league. My dad would always ask how her season was going. Seeing his interest and that of other residents, the facility arranged a trip to see one of the league's games. Even though they didn't stay for the entire game, my dad talked about it for over a year. This is an excellent example of a facility that responds to the individual residents' interests to make their day enjoyable and interesting, rather than monotonous.

WHAT WILL I EAT?

Meals are a prominent feature of any facility tour; however, you might underestimate how important they are to your loved one's comfort and well being. As his or her independence decreases, the structure of the day is often what he or she relies on. The three meals of the day can become the major milestones of the day and are the times when your loved one will likely spend the most time socializing with other residents. It is important that the food is of high quality and that he or she likes the food and the dining room atmosphere. Can your loved one order what he or she wants or are choices limited? Is the food familiar? Will he or she sit with other residents with whom they are comfortable?

If any of these details are unacceptable, your loved one will dislike the facility no matter how attractive other aspects are. For example, my dad's family was from Cornwall, England, where one of the common meals is a pasty, a very basic vegetable, potato, and meat pie. For him, food was simple and his only concept of a spice was ketchup. Therefore, the relatively spicy ethnic food served at his first facility was delicious for some residents, but for my dad it was a nightmare. He dropped twenty pounds within the first six months of moving in, a fact that contributed to us making the choice to move him to another facility.

You should also ask whether the residents are able to eat in their rooms. Facilities vary on this subject. Some do not allow meals to be served in residents' rooms, citing the need to keep rooms clean and to make sure the resident eats. They may also want to avoid allowing residents to stay by themselves in their rooms. However, other facilities will bring a food tray to the resident's room if requested. My dad liked to eat in his room when he was upset or feeling down. He simply wanted peanut butter and banana on toast in his room where it was peaceful. Again, a facility that will work with you to make your loved one comfortable is what you should look for.

If having his or her evening cocktail is important to your loved one, you should inquire about the facility's policy on alcohol. Many facilities do not offer alcohol and have strict policies about its consumption by residents. However, some will offer wine or a limited choice of other alcoholic beverages at the evening meal. Some facilities may even have small "cocktail parties" in the late afternoon in a common area where light beverages and snacks are served. Again, every facility is different.

Be sure to understand how seating arrangements are determined in the dining room. Can your loved one pick where he or she sits, or is seating assigned? If assigned, does the facility regularly change where your loved one sits? Also, can your loved one change his or her table if requested? For example, at his facility my dad sat with all the male residents (facilities often have more women than men). Unfortunately, several of the men at his table were experiencing early signs of dementia and could be very disruptive during dinner. No matter how good the food, the other residents asking the same questions over and over made my dad want to leave the table as soon as possible. We finally solved the problem by asking that he be moved to a table with other residents who had similar capabilities as him. Remember most residents (and your loved one) will change over time. You certainly cannot control all of these factors; but you want to make sure the facility will be open to work through problems and concerns if they arise.

Additionally, your loved one can easily become depressed when he or she first moves into an assisted living facility, and decreased appetite is often a common symptom. If they do not like the food, or the other residents at their table are disruptive, it will add to their lack of appetite. Therefore, meals are that much more of a deciding factor when selecting a facility.

SHOW ME MY ROOM

As you tour the facilities on your list, you and your loved one will see what types of rooms are available. Most have a variety of layouts that increase in size and cost. Some rooms are very simple, with only a bedroom and a bathroom. Others will also include a small kitchenette with a sink, refrigerator, and cupboards. Still others will resemble small apartments with a sitting room, bedroom and kitchenette. Also take into account whether or not your loved one will share a room, and if so, evaluate how the space is divided between the two residents. Will your loved one have sufficient privacy? If both your parents are moving, does the facility have specific accommodations for them as a couple? Will the facility allow them to live together if their abilities and medical needs are different?

When looking at bathrooms, see how easily your loved one can navigate them. Remember that you can add shower chairs and elevated toilet seats to make the bathroom more accessible.

If your loved one wants to bring a significant amount of belongings, particularly furniture, you will want to request the dimensions of rooms to determine which layout best fits their needs (or if your loved one must further pare down his or her belongings given the room size he or she can afford). It is also important to ask whether you can freely decorate the room, including painting it the color your loved one prefers. Know that anything you can do to help your loved one enjoy his or her new living arrangement will be worth it. For my dad, we filled the walls with his favorite family photos and quilts he had received as gifts. When we had to move to a different assisted living facility, we carefully took down the wall decorations and then reinstalled them in his new room in a way that helped make the move feel not as much of a change as it was.

Another important consideration is determining where your loved one's room will be located in relationship to staff work areas. If your loved one requires more care, it might be preferable to pick a room near the nurse's station, the front desk, or the elevator. You might want a centrally located room where staff regularly walking by and can easily check in on your loved one. If, alternatively, your loved one needs extra care and his or her room is removed from the heavy traffic areas, it will be harder for him or her to get needed attention without constantly ringing for staff. Obviously, you have to balance the need for staff access with the noise and disruption that may come from being in a more visible location.

Also, ask about controlling both heat and air conditioning. Is the temperature gauge in a location that is easily accessed by your loved one? If the room you are considering features many windows, check for drafts and secure shades so your loved one can keep the room at a comfortable temperature.

WHERE CAN I GO AND HOW DO I GET THERE?

Availability of transportation is always an important question to ask. Does the facility have its own van that can take residents to activities? For example, some facilities take residents to local churches on Sunday or on regular lunch outings at local restaurants. Is there transportation to medical appointments? If the facility does not have its own transportation, they may help schedule community senior transportation, which may be available in your area for a small fee. If your loved one uses a community bus, make sure you know if the bus driver will assist your loved one with getting on and off the bus and into their appointment.

Also, if your loved one still drives, find out if he or she can keep a car at the facility. Is the car parked inside or outside? My dad LOVED his car. Without it, he was lost, even long after he was unable to drive. The fact that we could keep his car in the facility's underground parking structure so my brother could take him for rides when he came home to visit made all the difference in his attitude toward his new living quarters. Our family also eventually hired a driver who took my dad in his car to church or to the park a few times a week. Having this option made my dad feel more independent and less confined.

WHAT OTHER SERVICES ARE OFFERED?

You should inquire what other services the facility offers that might be important to your loved one. Can your loved one bring his or her pet? Does the facility have its own therapy dog living at the facility? Does the facility offer cable TV? Is there an extra cost for that? Does the facility have wireless Internet? If not, can you install it in your loved one's room? Many seniors are becoming more computer literate so they can stay in touch with loved ones via email and social media. Even if your loved one is not interested in using the computer, having the Internet available makes connecting your loved one with far away relatives and friends that much easier for you. By using Skype to wish my dad a happy Father's Day as a family, we made the day that much more special for him.

Finally, consider whether the facility has classes that might interest your loved one. Do local musicians or choirs come to the facility to give concerts? If your loved one loves to plays music, does the facility have a piano? If your loved one enjoys bird watching or gardening, is there an outdoor space with bird feeders and gardens for him or her to enjoy? Can your loved one plant his or her own small garden? Anything that can add interest to your loved one's day is important to consider.

THE BOTTOM LINE...

- Determine what is the most convenient location for your loved one and you.

- Find out the facility's schedule. What is the flow of caregiving, meals, and activities?

- Know if residents and family can come and go from the facility at will.

- Make sure your loved one will eat the food served by the facility and that it meets his or her dietary needs.

- Understand how the facility organizes seating in the dining room, and if staff is flexible regarding it when necessary.

- Make sure your loved one can navigate the bathroom of his or her potential room.

- Ask for room dimensions to help in planning what belongings your loved one will bring.

- Ask about the facility's policies regarding painting and decorating your loved one's room.

- Consider where your loved one's room will be situated in relation to staff work stations.

- Find out the available transportation options at the facility.

- Consider other amenities and services the facility might offer, including classes and outdoor spaces.

10.

THINK "OUTSIDE THE BOX"

Before making a final decision about which assisted living facility to choose, take a moment to consider whether an assisted living facility is the best option. You now know a lot more about what assisted living facilities in your area have to offer and hopefully you've talked openly with your loved one and your family about the pros and cons of all of the choices. So now take a moment to ask: Is this the best option right now?

Consider the Alternatives to Assisted Living Facilities

Look again at the alternatives. For example, might it be better to have your loved one remain in their home but with in-home care? Examine the costs and see how they compare to assisted living facilities. Do you know another family facing the same decision for their loved one? Is it possible to move your loved ones into one home and share the cost of in-home care? Evaluate whether your loved one's insurance might pay for some of the in-home care. The federal government has recently made changes to the law, and it now allows seniors to use their insurance to pay for some of this care.

Can Your Loved One Live with a Caregiver?

Is it possible a family member or a college student could move in with your loved one to assist with care and be there during the night? Providing housing in exchange for some help for your loved one might work for everyone. You may still need some additional medical in-home care, but having someone you know living with your loved one helps you more easily monitor the care that is being given.

It might be an option to move your loved one into a smaller, ground floor apartment or condominium. This could allow your loved one to keep living independently, but they will have less upkeep and easier mobility as they age. Another option is to consider whether your loved one might enjoy being with different members of your family throughout the year. For example, if you and your loved one reside in a cold climate and you have a sibling in California, your loved one could live with him or her in the winter months. During the summer, he or she could live with you or another family member. Having this arrangement allows your loved one to live with family, but allows the burden of care to not fall to one person exclusively.

These are only some of the creative options to consider before moving to an assisted living facility. Yet, after considering all options, you and your loved one may still decide that assisted living is the best option for everyone. The more information you gather and the more discussion you and your loved have, the better the chances are that you will make the decision that is right for everyone, most importantly your loved one.

THE BOTTOM LINE...

- Think creatively before settling on assisted living as the right option for your loved one.

- Consider having your loved one remain in their home, but with additional in-home care.

- Consider having someone move in with your loved one to assist with care and provide companionship.

- Consider downsizing your loved one's housing.

- Consider having your loved one live with different family members throughout the year.

TERMS TO KNOW

Activities of Daily Living (ADLs): Aspects of daily life, such as dressing, bathing, going to the bathroom, taking medication, and eating that assisted living facilities help residents with. The cost of assisted living is often tied to the type and number of ADLs requiring assistance.

Aging in place: Approach to senior care that focuses on keeping a senior in one environment, such as a continuing care community, while adding services to meet his or her increasing needs as he or she ages.

Assisted living facility: Residential facility that assists seniors with aspects of daily living while focusing on providing as much independence as possible.

Caregiver: An individual, usually a family member, who provides non-professional care for a senior.

Continuing care retirement community: Facilities that provide graduated levels of care for seniors with varying needs and levels of autonomy. These facilities often feature privately owned homes for active seniors, an assisted living facility, and a skilled nursing home.

Durable power of attorney: A legal document that allows someone you designate to act on your behalf should you become incapacitated and cannot make decisions for yourself. Durable power of attorney allows that other person to make pay bills, write checks, and make other transactions on your behalf.

Independent living: Refers to seniors who live on their own in their own home or those who live in active adult communities and need little or no assistance with aspects of daily living.

In-home care: Care provided to seniors in their homes by family, friends, or professional aids.

Long term care insurance: Coverage that provides nursing home care, home healthcare, personal or adult day care for individuals over sixty five or who have a chronic and disabling condition that requires constant care.

Medicaid: A joint federal- and state-funded program that provides healthcare to low-income Americans.

Medical power of attorney: Legal document that allows someone you designate to make decisions regarding your healthcare and medical treatment when you cannot make decisions or cannot communicate your wishes regarding your care.

Medicare: Insurance program run by the federal government that provides health coverage to people over the age of sixty five. Medicare also provides coverage for people with certain disabilities as well as those with end stage renal disease.

Nursing home: Facility that provides comprehensive assistance with activities of daily living and continuous medical care.

Personal emergency alert device: A device worn as a necklace or bracelet that, when activated, alerts caregivers or emergency medical personnel that the wearer has experienced a medical emergency.

Rehabilitation facility: Facility where individuals recovering from serious injury or illness can receive intensive therapy to regain physical strength or rebuild skills such as speaking or walking.

Senior community: Large facility, such as an apartment complex, that houses seniors in an independent living setting.

LORI-ANN'S ON YOUR SIDE

"When I need health care advice I can understand and follow, I call Lori-Ann. She knows her stuff!"
M. Diane Vogt, JD

"Lori-Ann is my "go-to" expert on healthcare law. She makes it understandable and easy to follow for our doctors and their patients, too."
Michele Nichols, The Physician Alliance

"Lori-Ann knows the healthcare system inside and out. Whenever we have questions about healthcare, Lori-Ann has the answers."
Mike Gerstenlauer, St. John-Macomb Hospital

"Whenever my family has a health care issue, Lori-Ann is my first call for the best advice."
Donna Curran

"Getting coverage for prescription drugs can be a big problem for patients. Lori-Ann knows the insider secrets to making it easy."
Coreen Buehrer

"Lori-Ann has also lived the difficult issues that families confront on a daily basis as they struggle with the bewildering maze of hospitals, multiple specialists and insurance companies as our family's tireless advocate for our father. No mother grizzly ever fought for her cubs with more passion than Lori-Ann looked out for our dad."
Stephen Rickard, J.D., MPA

About the Author

Lori-Ann Rickard is one of the country's top healthcare lawyers. For over three decades, she has advised leading hospitals, doctors, laboratories, and other healthcare providers. Now she offers her expertise to patients and their families through the Easy Healthcare Series from HealthSpin.

Lori-Ann is also a single mom of two beautiful daughters. One of her daughters was very sick when she was born. Already caring for a toddler and managing a developing career, Lori-Ann used her professional experience to create quick, effective strategies to make the healthcare system work for her as she sought the best treatment possible for her sick baby. Later, Lori-Ann served as the primary caregiver and medical coordinator for her proud, independent parents when they became unable to care for themselves. Through their wellness challenges, her daughter's illness, and in helping friends over the past thirty years, Lori-Ann has used her unique position in the industry to create easy healthcare solutions that work for everyone around her. These solutions will work for you and your family, too.

Lori-Ann Rickard is a healthcare insider who knows what it means to be a patient and a caregiver. The Easy Healthcare Series brings you the benefit of Lori-Ann Rickard's expertise. Let her show you how you can Spin Your Healthcare Your Way.

More By Lori-Ann Rickard

Visit myhealthspin.com to download your free copy
of *Easy Healthcare: What You Need First!*
ALSO AVAILABLE FROM HEALTHSPIN:

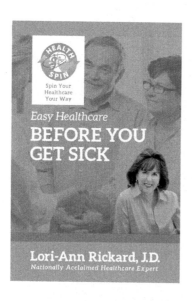

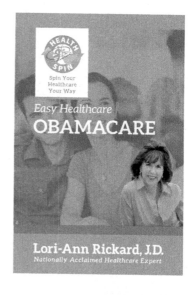

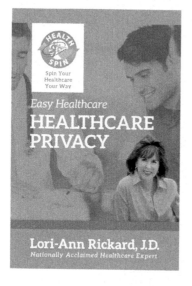

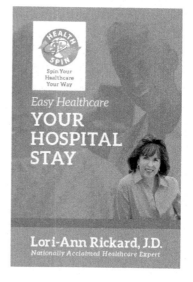

CPSIA information can be obtained
at www.ICGtesting.com
Printed in the USA
LVOW01s1611240317
528386LV00007B/633/P